Nursing Home Sweet Home

Nursing Home Sweet Home

Dr. Rod G. Bjordahl

VANTAGE PRESS
New York

Published by Vantage Press, Inc.
516 West 34th Street, New York, New York 10001

Manufactured in the United States of America
ISBN: 0-533-12175-2

Library of Congress Catalog Card No.: 96-90795

0 9 8 7 6 5 4 3 2 1

Contents

Preface

This collection of prose and poetry is in a sense a celebration of age and memories and joy within suffering. The various stories are summaries of feelings acquired during this physician's years of caring for residents in a nursing home. I always wanted to be an artist, but I couldn't draw, a definite setback in my career planning. When I see the beauty of happy and unhappy scenes or persons, the warmth and spirit of those things beg to be drawn, but I can't. Writing has been a way I can capture these feelings for myself so I don't lose them. I hope you enjoy these "drawings" in prose and poetry.

Activities

Activities at nursing homes are apparently meant to humor the old folks so they don't start a riot. At least that is my isolated opinion. Most of us don't complain when certain activities don't appeal to us. If we did, we would probably just get that "Oh, try it, you'll like it" garbage. Who can like cutting out snowflakes from construction paper or singing "God Bless America" when you're an atheist. How about those trips to the zoo when you get diarrhea from the spoiled mayonnaissed sandwich, or those cookie-baking sessions where the help eats all the cookies. The periodic outside entertainers are sometimes interesting. Last week we had a magician who somehow set fire to the stage curtains and we got to watch the fire department put it out. Now that was entertaining.

The activities I want to see are something like pin-the-tail-on-the-donkey or spin-the-bottle or gambling with real money. How about a burping contest or motorized wheelchair races? Or maybe next time they bake those cookies we can have a cookie-eating contest.

Airs of Joy

When I leave here
I will walk tall
My face into the winds
Of the past and future
My nostrils flaring
My lungs expanding
Under stretching ribs
To accept the airs of joy.

Anticipation

Perhaps sadness is what you see
When you look at me
That's what you asked
As you passed.

But it is not sadness for now,
For what can I do about it?
I am here to stay
No matter what anyone can say.

My expression mirrored my mind,
Which was visiting the past,
Dwelling on a moment to treasure
A time filled with pleasure.

The sadness was for what I missed
But I can't resist,
Grabbing at a past bliss
To cover the unpleasantness of all this.

This now is my aged time
Well past the years golden
Waiting in happy anticipation
For my eternal vacation.

Aware

Thanks for the touch;
It's something I miss so much.

It makes me feel you care
That of me you are aware.

Beyond the White Light

I just had to write
To let you know
I'm all right
I transcended peacefully
The other night.
You must have heard
The word
By now.

It was similar
To the books written
By those returned
But no authors
Had yet been past
The white door
Before
'til now.

There was first pain
Then no pain
Then tunnels
From dark to light
Focusing me
Like wind
To forward
Destiny.

Then the threshold
To the beyond
Past the light
It became expansive

Yet personal
I was me
And Thee

And we.

All to see
Words unknown
Atoms first seen
Smells never smelled
Familiar yet
New eyes looked
New suns shown
Flights taken
Loves unshaken.

All wrongs were right
Chaos was sense
Recall was total
Futures seen
Were now and past
Slow was fast
First was last
Evil avast.

Old concerns have left
You will see soon
Time is unknown
My so-called life
An instant
I watch now pass
Ever so fast
And infrequent.

All that ever was
And shall ever be
I have seen
All who ever were
And ever shall be
Is here and neat
All at peace with
Jobs complete.

There are no doubts
No forms unfamiliar
Spirits are one
Equal to all
Sweet within
Moving as willed
Even those
Who have killed.

Telling you this
Is no need,
For as you are there
You are here
Saying my same words
Thinking my same thoughts,
For all are one
Now, then and when.

So beyond the white light
Your words cannot
Your there-mind cannot
Explain or know or say,
For that truth
Can be seen only
By what is seen
With no in-between.

Feel no agony or loneliness
Fear not your own death
Fear not your mistakes
For since conception
To transcention
We had the promise that
All spirits will receive this
Their eternal bliss.

Birth Announcements

Jeffrey and Nona Estness, Evansville, are the parents of their first son, Jonathan, born November 19th. He weighed 8 lbs. and measured 22 inches.

Grandparents of the newborn are Frederick and Mary Volker and Arnold and Ginger Estness, all of Evansville.

Great-Grandmother is Marie Martha Estness, currently residing in Northville Nursing Home in Evansville.

Characters

We have quite a few characters here on our wing. Actually, most of them are characters. I guess if you live long enough you will become a character. Or is that you have to be a character to live long?

For example, old Nathan down in Room 103 was a fighter pilot in World War II. He has Alzheimer's now. The only thing that will get him out of an agitated time is if you call him "Major" and salute him. It quiets him right down. Better than drugs, the nurses say.

Herbert is pretty cool, too. He was in a helicopter that crashed in a volcano. He had some major head injury, so now he is totally paralyzed and can't talk. He can blink his eyes for "yes" and not blink his eyes for "no" and he is an avid television sports fan. You can go down there to his room and tell him who are the final four at any playoff sport and he can pick the final winner. You just have to ask him "yes" or "no" questions and he will blink out the answer like a computer. We have made a few small bets on his predictions and won easily. Everyone asks how we pick the winners. We don't tell them.

Mr. Domingo is our weather man. His arthritis is the type such that he will start to have joint pains about twenty four hours before its rains. If we have an outing planned, we will ask him first if it is going to be rainy that next day and if he hurts, we stay home and play bingo. He has better predicting ability that the television weather man.

Marilyn is a real trip. Even at her advanced age of eighty-eight, she still has the sex drive of a thirty-year old. She too is bedridden, but when she sees a man walk by outside the door, she beckons him with her index finger and warbles a cute: "Yoo-hoo, yoo-hoo." Some of the men go in to see her and they hold hands and say sweet things to each other for a while and then they depart looking very much happier. Ah, those were the good old days.

Me? Nothing special. I don't feel as though I am a character really. But I sure like to watch and listen and imagine what these fellow residents were like in their younger years. We all sure had a good time.

Comfortable Struggle

To dream while awake
Is a gift at times
An escape from my pain
And even from my shame.

I look only straight ahead
To avoid seeing my body
Once a thing of beauty
Staying now only out of duty.

This indulgence won't last, don't leave,
I sink here every now
And then I return
To thoughts that don't burn.

One needs to mind move
To shift from the repulsive
To the inner theatre place
Of fiction, myth and grace.

The young body strong did speed
Ahead of the then-empty mind
Only to later have aged body need
The full-knowing mind to heed.

It tells me now it is good
To have this nursing home sweet
Home of my last bed
To comfort my struggle to meet those dead.

Conversational Thought

Ah, here comes my doctor to make his regular visit.

"Good morning, Mrs. Johnson, how are we today?"

The morning looks fine, bozo, and you know I can't answer you since I had my stroke. And who is the "we" . . . I am only one person here.

"Looks like we are going to finally get that rain we needed."

What would dense people ever do without the weather?

"Are they feeding you okay here?"

The food tastes like shit and I don't have any teeth to chew anyway.

"I noticed from your medical chart that you are having regular bowel movements."

Sure, if you think a bowel movement every morning at five o'clock when you don't get up until seven o'clock is "regular."

"Now let me check your heart and lungs and see how they are doing."

They are doing terrible and I'm sure he is going to say that my lungs are filling okay and my heart is a good strong heart.

"Well, your lungs are filling okay and your heart is a good strong heart."

Boring.

"Well, Mrs. Johnson, I'm going to the nurses' station and renew your orders. Do you need anything else?"

Sure, Doctor, if you can read my mind, order me a six-pack of beer and a deck of cards so I can feel human again.

"See you next month, Mrs. Johnson. Take care."

Come back again, Doc. I really do enjoy these visits.

Disjointed Mental Movies

John Wayne had a walk
Tough guy walk of the West.
What's that song?
Old-time song and dance.
A beauty she was
Just because.

What are you looking at?
Troubled eyes get away
Should I be afraid?
I am afraid
Danger, danger,
I see a stranger.

Baseball, get outa my room
Smell the dirt
Walk out there
You can do it
I remember I did
I remember I did.

Left foot, right foot
Left foot, right foot
Right foot, right foot
Right foot, wrong foot
Kick the can
If you can.

Hello, where's my brother?
Just saw him there
Dead long time say you
You're wrong
Don't like you
I'll find him, you'll see.

New people every day
Don't know many
Used to know everyone
World has changed
New owners, I guess
Gone out farther west.

Don't Judge Me

Please don't judge me by my feet. God, are they ugly. Why are feet so unattractive compared to hands? Hands have character, like the face. Remember all of those "thinking" photographs where the hands are held thoughtfully against the chin. Have you ever seen such a photograph with the person's foot against his chin?

Feet are so characterless. They all seem grotesque and not nearly as nice as the people they move around. It probably has something to do with gravity and all those years of carrying that weight around. Hands don't carry weight around, that's why they look so nice. Feet don't look friendly even when the person may be friendly. Feet look tired and fussy and left out. Maybe they get that way because they are the last to get blood.

Look at my feet, they're old and awful. I can't stand them either. How many people do you know of who really like their feet? If they say they like them, they probably are in denial.

Even Though

Listen to me even though I
    Cannot speak

See me even though you
    Cannot bear to

Help me even though my needs you
    Cannot know

Understand me even though our minds
    Cannot meet

Let me go even though this wish you
    Cannot understand

Remember me even though I understand you
    Cannot.

I Am Fine

Being by myself and being quiet by myself is not a bad thing. Too often the nurses come by and ask how I am. I say I am fine. Their faces then show that sweet concern that seems to say I am probably not telling the truth.

But I am okay. My roommate and I rarely converse with each other even though we have lived together in the same room for seven years. She's a dear. I'm a dear too, or so they say. We both do so enjoy our solitude.

We really aren't sad or depressed or demented. This is just our life, for as long as we have it. Life at our age and in this nursing home is our way now. One place is no different from another, no better or worse than another. It is curiously like another dimension in another time or another universe.

There are glimpses of the prior world from time to time, but they are short in duration and only vaguely familiar and only vaguely pleasant. What was so vital then is not vital now. What is vital now might not be vital tomorrow. Being is vital. If I am not here tomorrow, that is okay and is also vital. We don't sit and wish for visitors. We don't sit and wish for anything that isn't here now.

As things change and new persons arrive and grow up and grow older, time passage itself becomes the most intriguing thing I contemplate in my solitude. Solitude and silence and time are all siblings in my family of life and living.

We all get along so well.

I Feel Good

Gosh, today I feel so good
One of those days rare
When my body seems silent
To the diseases residing there.

These days are nice
They are like gifts sweet
Like promises of my end
When life's problems will sleep.

I'm Sorry, So Sorry

I wonder why that old song keeps coming back to me? Something like, "I'm sorry, so sorry, that I was such a fool." Do I really feel sorry? I don't feel sorry for now or for myself. Who sang that song anyway?

When I look at young folks, I feel sorry for them when they will no longer be young. When I see old folks like me, I feel sorry for them but not for me. Strange.

When I saw the new patient with the half-paralyzed body, I felt sorry that he may not have done all he wanted to do before his stroke. I want to apologize to him, for not telling him before that he might have a stroke, but I didn't and don't even know him. Strange.

Was I "such a fool?" I didn't think I was then, but now I think I was then. To have raced through life with such unobservant recklessness, I must have been a fool. To have hurt so many people and not later apologized. I must have been a fool to have destroyed this body so, to have not given a damn so many times. I must have been a fool. But that's what life is, they say. Live it to the fullest. Too often that means to live life to the reckless fullest.

It would be nice now to have walked ten miles through the Wisconsin farmlands that summer instead of the three miles I did. I should have lain on my back in that meadow flower field for six hours instead of ten minutes. How nice the earth felt, so unbelievably warm and familiar. Strange, but not strange.

Connie Frances! That's who sang that song. Beautiful.

It's Not Fair

I have tried so hard
To understand what life is
What existence is
What being is
But at my last days
I am still lost.

It's not fair
To study mathematics
Physics, art, chemistry
Medicine and what all
And still not know
Why I am still lost?

What sense to be born
To live such a long life
To travel and love
And drink to drunk
And smoke to choke
And yet be lost.

What twisted mind
Would dream such a torture
To set us out alone
Slap us around and wrinkle us
Give us fear and disease and regret
Then keep the reason for it secret.

Leave Me Alone

Leave me alone
Distance from you I need
Younger thought
Doesn't mix with older.

Your words like dribble
Chatter without direction
Do others listen to this?

My young words
Had more feeling
More sense to them
Back then.

I can move my attention
And your words become
Like distant gnats
That I swat from my ears.

How dumb you are
Your annoyance
Makes me tired
Go away
Leave me alone.

Like Superman Flying

I had that dream again last night, the one about seeing my mother in the white gown flying through the air. I understand it more now. The first time was right after she died forty-five years ago. It scared me then, but now I even look forward to it. It's a peaceful work of art now.

The dream starts with her cruising up to me like Superman flying through the clouds. She looks so peaceful. At first I was shocked because she looked unexpectedly good for a dead person. Then she says she loves me and that I shouldn't worry because she is just fine. She tells me that I could join her right now if I wanted to, but it's okay to wait because she will always be there no matter when I come. Then she gives me that loving look and glides on her way.

Love Note First

Dear Arthur,

Please excuse my penmanship. I have a little tremor problem. I used to have the nicest penmanship.

I asked the nurse to slip you this note because I just had to tell you something. Ever since seeing you at bingo last Friday in the activity room, I have had an upset stomach. No, I'm not sick. That's the way I get when I am strongly attracted to a handsome gentleman like you.

If you feel the same, please send me a note. Use Nurse Nicole to send it. . . . She's nice.

Cordially yours,
Myrtle Olson

Love Note Two

Dear Myrtle,

I think your handwriting is just fine.
This is Arthur.
I got your note. Can I sit with you at bingo Friday night?

Sincerely,
Arthur Johnson
Room 103A

Love Note Three

Dear Arthur,

I so enjoyed sitting at bingo with you last night. You're even cuter up close. Were you wearing Old Spice or Coppertone? I love them both. I mean, I love them both on you.

Thank you for giving me your winning card. I never won anything before.

Wonderful night. Sort of chilly. Your arm kept me warm. You still have nice big arms.

Love,
Myrtle

Love Note Four

Dear Myrtle,

   I think I caught your upset stomach. Never thought of falling in love at this age. I don't like that word "falling" in a nursing home. Too many folks go out that way.
   Myrtle, don't you go out now that I have found you.
   Thanks for the cookies.

Love,
Arthur

Love Note Five

Dearest Arthur,

These last six months have been lovely, haven't they? I don't think I have ever been happier. You're such a nice lover.

Nicole told me you were doing time at the hospital and that your hip was healing fine. I guess you had that fall you were worried about. And on the way to my room, too. How sweet.

Please write.

Love you forever,
Myrtle

Love Note Six

Dear Myrtle,

Boy, do I miss my sweet cheeks, Myrtle.
This hospital is nice, but without you it's hell.
The doctor says next week I can return if everything
is okay.

See you, honey,
King Arthur

Love Note Last

My Arthur,

I feel funny writing to you when you're not with us but just one more note before I see you next.

Sorry to hear you died. Sorry for me because I am lonely without you. You always did want to lead the way with me, didn't you?

Nicole was a little puzzled that I wasn't more sad when she told me. She'll understand some day.

Keep those big arms open for me. See you soon.

Eternally,
Myrtle

Mother Visits Home

I hadn't been downtown or back to my old home in a long time. The last time was about five years ago. Things happen you know.

There were the two trips to the hospital for my heart failure and then my daughter died. Before you knew it, five big ones went by.

It's like that in nursing homes. Not as boring as you might think. Someone always coming or going, most of them with no choice in the matter, of coming or going, I mean.

But, here I am, cruising down Main Street in my son's van. He had to buy the van for me and his kids. Me for my wheelchair and for his kids he just needed some distance between them and the back of his head. Kids can be the most uncoordinated living things on the earth, but they can hit the back of the head of their father in the driver's seat from thirty yards out with just about any disgusting object.

Boy, the downtown sure seems different. I swear it looks faded, just like an old photograph. The buildings look the same, except the corners and middles seem droopy. I should holler. You ought to see my corners and middle.

But true, they do seem somewhat tired. Imagine carrying all those people and groceries and beds around inside of you for decades after decades. Who wouldn't look tired. Some of them look like they are going to collapse and split out at their stretch marks. Don't say it.

There's the Piggly Wiggly grocery store. I remember Mom going in there. While she was buying the potatoes and pear and pork, I was snitching the peanuts and pop.

Later on I ended up being a cashier there. The place seems like one of the family.

Well, I'll be. That sure looks like Ole Olson standing there outside Rorge's Bar. But he's supposed to be my age. I must be having a flashback or a hot flash. Don't I wish. My son says that's Ole's son. Like father, like son, they say. My son also says he was appropriately named Ole junior. Good grief. Midwestern brain storm ideas, what insight, what ingenuity. "Let's name him Ole, honey." Now, there he is, carrying on the family tradition, helping to keep the wall of Rorge's Bar from falling into the street. Somebody has to do it, I guess.

Churches and bars, churches and bars, the mainstay of the Main Street at the Midwest. A lot of comfort in that, I guess. You need money for both, so it keeps the boys working. The ladies just have to get their household money from the blue jeans at night. The men never miss it. They're on a run, on a path, on a goal, so they don't miss what is lost along the way.

Good men, though. Good places, good streets, good buildings, good memories. Well, there's my old house. Looks nice. Looks the same. Doesn't look faded. Can't believe I'm crying like a baby.

Nature

Nature seems different to me now when I am not so young.

When I was a child, nature surprised me, scared me, baffled me. Thunder was frightening, darkness was death, but snow was so beautiful.

Then as a non-old adult, it was my duty to conquer Nature, to keep the rain out, to protect my children from the thunder, and to move snow out of my living space. The snow was still beautiful.

Now at my older age, Nature has stopped being so remote. Nature is my friendly companion, my equal, my spirit guide, so to speak. I love its smells, its loudness, its music. I now love that which I feared and thought I conquered.

And, oh my, the snow is still so beautiful.

Obituaries

Marie Martha Estness, 89, Evansville, died at 7:15 P.M. on November 19th at Northville Nursing Home.

She was born January 19, 1906 in Evansville and lived her entire life there. She married Olaf Estness in 1930, who preceded her in death 12 years ago. Mrs. Estness and her husband maintained the family farm until 12 years ago when the reins were taken by their son Arnold. Marie was locally famous for rhubarb pie and her many card party championships.

Services will be held this Sunday at 11:00 P.M. at the Woodhill Lutheran Church. Potluck lunch will follow.

Old Folks Don't Cry Much

Ever notice
Old folks don't cry much
How come
Why won't they
Why don't they
Don't they feel
Aren't they sad
Don't they care
Don't they dare
Are they numb
Are they dumb
They eat and
They sleep
They yell
They sit a long spell
But they don't cry much
Ever notice
Even in pain
Even with death
Even with nothing
Unable to sing
Unable to drive
Unable to run
Never much fun
Even with all this
Old folks don't cry much
Ever notice.

Popo

"Popo" is all that comes out
A native word for grandma
I think of other words to say
But my only sentence stays as "Popo."

I loved her so when she was here
Always so warm and huggy
Smelling sweet, singing soft to me
My ear to her chest heard beats saying, "Popo, Popo."

She died when I was young
Her age old like mine now
How empty and hurt I was then
To know I would not see again my "Popo."

Frustrating that my brain stroke
Stops me from making many words
But pleasing that the one name I miss
Remains on my lips like a kiss as "Popo."

Quiet All Day

Quiet all day am I
The choice though not mine,
Confined with brain loss, they say
Some vessel stopped feeding the mind.

Your fear uncertain is first seen
When on my presence you stare,
Wondering what am I and
What to say to me you dare?

Ah, but still I think
Still I know, I know more now
Than before, for more time
To ponder and wonder how.

Funny to see you looking sad
At my distorted form, for I see
More sadness in me for you
Seeking still life's superficiality.

So worry not, pity not, quit not
For as this outer form wilted,
Again though no choice of mine own,
Forgotten inner eternities became my new home.

(Reprinted by permission from *Poetic Voices of America,* Spring 1991. Sparrowgrass Poetry Forum, Sistersville, West Virginia.)

Rain

Too stupid to come in
Out of the rain
My parents told me
So in I would flee.

Cheated I felt
So much rain missed running
Licking water from lips
Imagining being at sea in ships.

Now I look out at storms
Unable to move lying still
Inhaling smells of weather rain
Dreaming only of being wet again.

Scared the Hell out of Me

Scared the hell out of me
It really did
There ought to be a law
Against those on the wall.

Hadn't seen one for years
Just been placed there
Some misguided do-gooder
Didn't like the wall bare.

Looked like a ghoul or beast
What a rush of fear
Thought I was a goner
Just me in that mirror.

She Said, He Said

"Please stop and talk to me. Yes, you. Oh, thank you so much," she said.

"Is there something wrong?" he said.

"No, I'm okay. I'm blind and my thin old bones keep me in bed, but I'm okay."

"Is there something I can do for you?"

"You already are. You see, my vision and body are gone, but my mind is still very good. It was one of my greatest things and now it is my only thing. All my life I thrived on conversation and intellectual exchanges. Now, that is all I have. If I do not continue to think and talk of stimulating, challenging things, I truly believe I will die."

"You shouldn't worry. You seem fine," he said.

"But you see, this mental activity is my life essence and my need for it is frighteningly overwhelming. I'm not sure how long I could go without it before I would die."

"How long have you gone in the past?" he asked.

"Once I got depressed and went for two months. They even gave me last rites. They had no idea what was wrong with me. You wouldn't believe all of the tests they did. Finally, I had to start conversing with just about anyone to come out of it. I had to before all those tests and medicines killed me," she answered.

"I see. I certainly would be happy to come by and talk from time to time. Maybe I could bring a book and read to you also, because I don't think my mind can keep up with yours all by itself," he said.

"Oh, that would be divine. You are so sweet! Will I see you next week then?" she asked.

"Yes, next week. Bye now," he said.

As he walked away, the charge nurse approached him.

"Hello, how are you tonight?" she said.

"Hello, Emma, I'm fine."

"How is your mother? Did she know you tonight?"

"No, not tonight, but the talking does seem to make her more energetic. It's hard still when she doesn't know me. But I guess I should be happy she hasn't left us yet."

"Yes, I guess so. If she knew you, she would be proud that you are her son. Will we see you again soon?" she asked.

"Yes, thank you again," he said.

"Good night, Doctor," she said.

Sundowning

Most of the daytime is okay here at the nursing home. My family said they were going nuts at home because I was going nuts. Now I'm here still going nuts, but going nuts is worse than not being nuts or being completely nuts. The difference is that you know the difference.

We have this thing called "sundowners" here. Daytimes are okay because days are new and promising and fresh like being born again. The night and the approaching night are not so optimistic. They are like death, like oversville, like slam-the-door-in-your-face, like remove your mailbox, like no place to sleep anymore, like kaput, the end, so long, sucker.

Now my early evenings are really wild. Just when the sun drops, I get these weird movies in my mind. Sure I know I have dementia, but I can take most of it in the daytime. I can just cover up the mistakes and people will usually just nod their heads and look dorky and I'm okay. But at sundown I see these bizarre movies and it seems I can play a part in any one of them if I just want to. No one seems to understand me when I do this. They look and listen and say, "He's just sundowning," and they go away.

Hey, I'm not sundowning! I have a problem. I can't decide which movie to be in and the indecisiveness is driving me nuts. I can't wait until I cross over into complete nutsville. Then I will be in only one movie and I will know the whole plot and I will know the ending and no one will be the wiser.

The Dinner Meeting

Ah, the old dinner crowd is here. The crowd is good, the food is good, the humor is good. Nursing home meals are a blast. Old folks have more fun than anyone else at mealtime. Why? Because, that's why, just because.

There goes Melvin dropping his spoon just when that cute nurse's aide comes by. He really likes her. It makes his whole day just to have her in his field of vision a few extra seconds. If your field of vision isn't what it used to be, you better fill it with pleasant-looking things for as long as you can.

Josephine likes to poke the jello and she smiles when it jiggles. She doesn't like it when they mix in the fruit cocktail because it cuts down on the jiggle time. Plus, jello is something you can stare into like a diamond or a crystal. Real exciting stuff for Josephine, the old jello crystal ball fortune teller.

Then there's Mandus, the mashed potato champ. He likes to put the mashed potatoes in his mouth, swallow some of it, and squirt the rest through his left five teeth out onto his chin. You ought to see that smile. He then laughs so hard at himself that he farts and then the farts get him laughing even more. Sometimes they just have to take him back to his room laughing potatoes all over and farting down the hallway.

Peas are good fun, especially for those old-timers who still insist on eating them off a knife. Let's not even mention the biscuit-throwing contests or the milk-out-the-nose trick.

I never knew how much fun dinner could be until I came to this wonderful nursing home.

The Girl and the Boy

She sits before me sobbing
Shakily telling me her loss,
Her eyes puffy and red
A tale of a lover long dead.

Wartime brave aviator he was
Tenderly strong face, moved with grace.
Together they were as one
Love vows under moon and sun.

He knew she knew war's risk
They looked them through like glass.
Thousands of miles of sea apart
He yet was there at her heart.

Then why for what end it came
Cold news of battle loss death.
A casualty, a number, a sorrow
She wished her death too tomorrow.

Have fifty years passed now lost?
Dutiful, numb, dispassionate voids.
Sweetly sparked by moments of joy
Those memories of the girl and the boy.

She cries now for to tell secrets all
Is to let him fully back to her.
Happily she finds his memory is he
And through eternity they are to be.

The One

Diane Anderson, the charge nurse on the Oakwood Wing at the nursing home, was soon to be married. She was in love but was having some pre-marital doubts. The major problem for her was that she wasn't sure if her future husband was "The One."

You know those stories about people saying, "Is he the one?" or "There's only one for you and when you find him, you'll know." But Diane was skeptical. How do you know? How do you know when to stop looking? Maybe there is a better "one."

Diane had the solution. To find out how to solve this problem, she was going to ask someone who had married only once and lived their entire life with one man. Certainly if you lived your whole life with someone, that someone had to be "The One."

As it was a small nursing home, it did not take Diane long to find Mary Stenson. She was 89 years old and her husband George had just passed away and she herself was apparently and rapidly on her way to join him. Mary would be the perfect expert.

"Mrs. Stenson, may I ask you a personal question?"

"Why, yes, you certainly can," replied Mary.

"Well, I am about to get married and I want to be sure my future husband is the right one. I want to know if he is the one and only one meant for me. I know that you were with one man all of your life, so you must have known how to decide who was the only one for you. So, I was hoping you could tell me how a girl picks or knows which man is the one meant for her. If I know how that is done, then I will know if I should get married now. Can you help me?"

Mary Stenson had been listening intently to the nurse

and was not at all surprised at the question. She herself had the same dilemma 70 years ago when she was to marry. *Amazing how some things don't change*, she thought. Here is this lovely, bright-eyed girl about to embark on the love journey and the same precious feelings that Mary had had were repeating themselves here again in this nurse, soon-to-be-wife.

"Honey, you bring up one of the great mysteries of life," answered Mary. "When we first fall in love, we feel that there is only one and for most it is. We are caught up, blinded, swept away, even want to die because nothing in the future could be better. I can see you feel that way now."

"So then is he the one, because I feel this way? Can I stop searching for any other because there is no other?" asked Diane.

"The mystery is also the myth," continued Mary. "Sure I was with only one man all my life and he was with only me. But I found out that that is only one way that companionship can be. All ways are essentially the one and the right way."

"Now, I'm really confused. At first you say my man is the one and then you say it's okay that he may not be? Can you please explain it more?"

"Yes, I think so," continued Mary. "You see, in life individuality many times is overdone. We are so alike in so many ways that we are almost one, all of us. So to say someone is the best or someone is prettier or someone is smarter is not necessarily something we need to do. If mankind is smart, then all of mankind plays some role in that smartness. If one person is said to be pretty, then all persons can be said to be pretty in some way. Are you following me so far?"

"Yes, maybe. Are you saying my fiancé is everyone?" inquired Diane.

"Essentially that is true," Mary said, looking strangely peaceful for some reason. "When you love one, you love all. Love whom you love, love deeply, and you are loving all. Loving one or just loving is loving existence, is loving every living thing. It is like a celebration every moment of your life, so you don't need to look beyond the love of the one, for it is the love of all."

Diane flushed over with some sort of energy surge and warmth and she wasn't sure why. But what Mary said touched something vital or spiritual in her, some type of fogged window cleared.

"Are you all right?" asked Mary. "Your colors are changing."

"Yes, Mary, I feel very fine. As a matter of fact, I feel great!"

"So what is your plan? With your fiancé I mean? What have you decided?" questioned Mary. "Is he the one?"

"Oh yes, most definitely, he is the one!"

The Underworld

Now that I have the time to, I enjoy watching small things. Their details are so amazing. Before my advanced age arrived, such details had no interest. I saw lawns of grass and not blades of grass.

For hours I can be perfectly still, bending over in my chair, watching insects, boulders of dust and such. What a fascinating world was being missed. I am able to mentally transport myself to that miniature world of the underworld, and explore all as I never thought possible before.

It is nice to know now of these other worlds since this body cannot travel the usual places it did so many decades ago.

It is very nice.

The Visit

Wow, lots of visitors today. I always worry when more family members visit me here at the home. If I was feeling really sick, I guess it would be normal. Let's have one more look at the old geezer before the grim reaper comes. But today I feel pretty good. Oh, oh, I remember those old movies where if you got shot and you had no pain, you were on the way to the hereafter. Nah, that can't be. I really do feel good and I don't see any blood.

So why are they here? Let's see. . . . Is it someone's birthday? Did my son get divorced again? Is my grand-daughter pregnant? Are my kids trying to make their kids respect old age?

Well, regardless, let's enjoy it anyway. Maybe they brought some Mogen David wine. Those nice nurses just cleaned me up, so I'm looking pretty good. I hope they're not going to tell me another friend of mine died. No, they aren't. This is looking more like a spur-of-the-moment visit. That's nice. I don't like events anymore anyway.

These, My Old Hands

Just look at them
These, my old hands,
Like stories in themselves
Like aged furrows of lands.

Out on the finger ends are
Knots of joints worked too much,
Hiding the now soft tips
Quietly recalling what they did touch.

Palms that used to callous hard
And help lift all in their way,
Now seem softly infantile
Wanting less to work than to play.

On top large vessels bulge
Circulating life's blood to places
That no longer seem needy,
But do anyway out of habit's graces.

The Pain

Oh, Lordy, here it comes again and it's a whopper this time. Smack dab in the middle of my chest, going to the left arm, making me gasp, making me sweat. Hard to believe you can sweat so much when you're just lying around doing nothing and it's almost freezing outside this time of year.

There, the nurse just brought me the nitroglycerin and put it under my tongue. It's amazing they treat this with explosives. I'm glad I don't have to swallow a stick of dynamite. Taking nitroglycerin sounds counterproductive at first speak.

I wonder if this is it, sure feels like it. Sort of like Jackie Gleason sitting on my chest, and maybe even Art Carney sitting on him. Holy smokes, Jesus, this is it, here I come. The pain is still climbing. I hope the grandchildren get a good education.

Ya, ya. I've already seen my whole life go by me many times before. I don't want to see it again. It was a boring movie the last few times. Besides, this time I think I know the ending. I hope I have some big bills outstanding. No more worries. No more problems. No more bozos. Goodbye, cruel world. I wonder if I'll kick my legs at the end? Why am I laughing?

Well, there it goes. No, not me, the pain. Tonight's not the night, I guess. I feel much better now, I can breathe. No sweats. Maybe there's something on television. Maybe I'll have a good night's sleep or even a visitor.

Time Goes By

Time goes by
So slowly
Yet at times
Looking back
It went so fast.

Can't remember
All that I thought
Or did
During that time
But so what.

I'm not sad
Just amazed
At my current
Indifference to time
And to thought.

These things were
So important before
And now I don't
Seem to care about them
Nor care to care.

Does that mean
I'm bad
To not care?
I don't think so
It feels fine.

Why is everything
So okay
When before
Everything
Never was just right.

Age and advanced
Maturity, I say,
Have their subtle
Advantages,
Don't they.

What to Miss

What does he miss?
I wonder to myself.
Wheelchair bound is he
Can't eat by himself either,
Wears a diaper under his clothes
Not so fun at eighty-one.

I would guess
He would miss running
Or driving or dancing.
Perhaps even football
Or baseball or hiking
Or dating or mating.

I asked him . . .
He thought, he sighed,
He smiled, he teared.
He surprised me, left me in awe,
Saying, "Doing a hard day's work
Is what I miss most of all. "